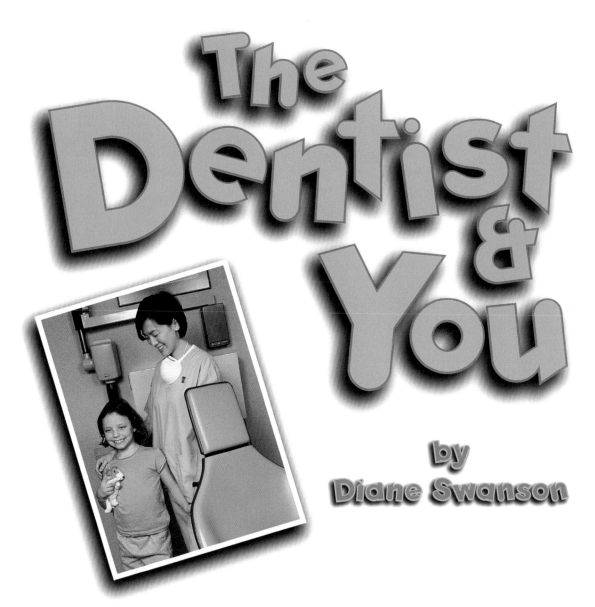

The Dentist & You

by Diane Swanson

ANNICK PRESS

TORONTO + NEW YORK + VANCOUVER

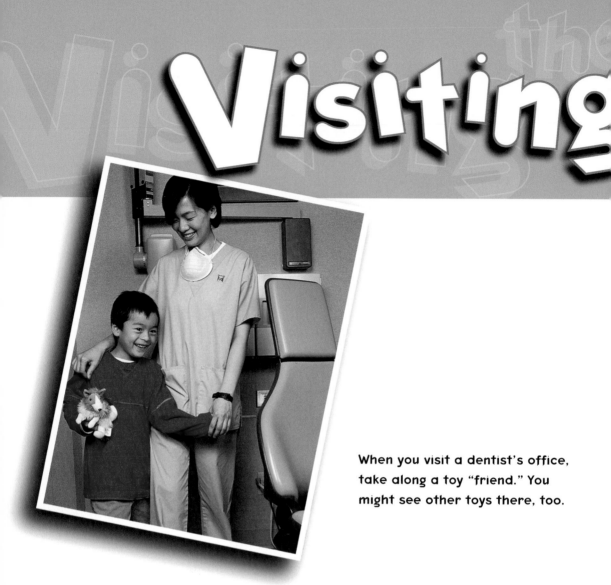

When you visit a dentist's office, take along a toy "friend." You might see other toys there, too.

Step up to a mirror and **SMiLE**. You're looking at a marvelous set of teeth. They help you chew your meals, speak clearly — even look great.

Every day, you protect your teeth by cleaning them. But like everybody else, you need a little help — at least twice a year. That's why you visit dentists regularly: to make sure you're cleaning all your teeth well and to prevent or fix problems.

the Dentist

Visiting dentists means going to offices that have special tools to care for your teeth. The dentists use many of them. Dental hygienists use some, too. The tools that are pictured in this book are common ones. You'll spot a lot of them on your visits — even if the tools don't look exactly like the ones on these pages.

When you see, hear, or feel a dentist's tools, they can seem strange. That's why it's good to read this book with a parent before you visit a dentist. You'll find out how the tools are used and why. You'll discover that most of them won't bother you at all and that a few might — just for a short time. But remember: these tools are there to help you.

You are the person in charge of your teeth, so you are important to their care. In this book, you'll read about some of the jobs you'll have at the dentist's office. Look for them on pages that say "Your Job." Then try them out on your dentist visits.

Seeing You Best

Try letting a friend or parent look at your teeth. You have to tip your head way back to show off all of them. That's tiring, so it's a good thing dentist offices have special chairs for checking teeth. The chairs have places to rest your head. And they can be leaned backward or forward—and raised or lowered. They make it easier for a dentist to examine your teeth and keep you comfortable.

Even when your mouth is open really **WIDE**, it's dark in some parts. That's why dentists and hygienists shine a bright light in there. They can move the lamp easily because it's on a metal arm that swings up, down, and around.

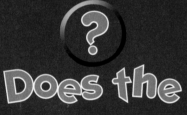

Does the Light Bother Your Eyes?

No. It's very bright, but it's angled so it doesn't hit your eyes. You might also be given some fun sunglasses to wear.

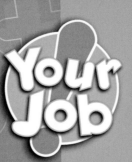

Your Job

Tell the dentist or hygienist if you feel uncomfortable in any way.

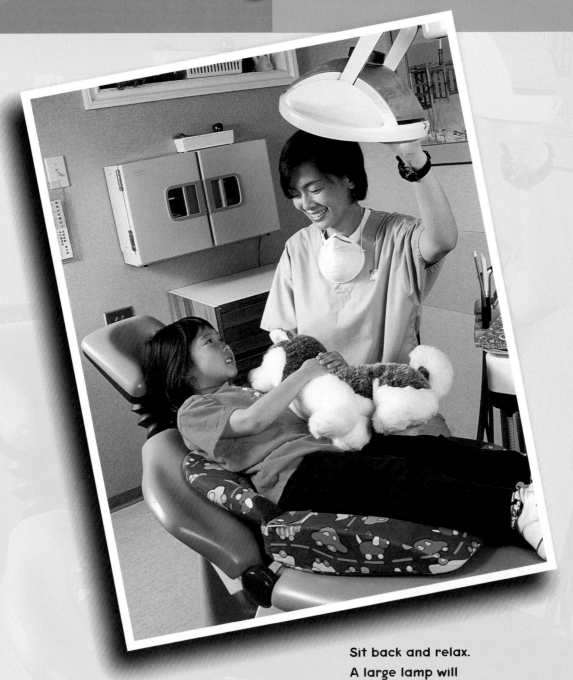

Sit back and relax. A large lamp will light up your mouth.

Dressed for the Job

A fun T-shirt, your favorite vest— even a Batman suit. Wear whatever you like to a dentist's office. But you probably want to keep your clothes clean and dry. That's why a large paper or plastic napkin is clipped under your chin when you sit in the dentist's chair. It's sometimes called a bib, but this is no baby's bib. Adults use the same kind.

Many dentists and hygienists wear uniforms. While they're working, they also cover their mouths and noses with masks and put on rubber gloves. They don't want to give you any of their germs—or get yours.

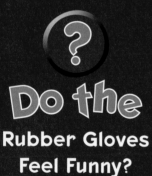

Do the Rubber Gloves Feel Funny?

The rubber is so thin you can barely feel the gloves when they touch your mouth.

Masks hide the smiling mouths of dentists and hygienists—but watch their eyes. You can see the smiles there.

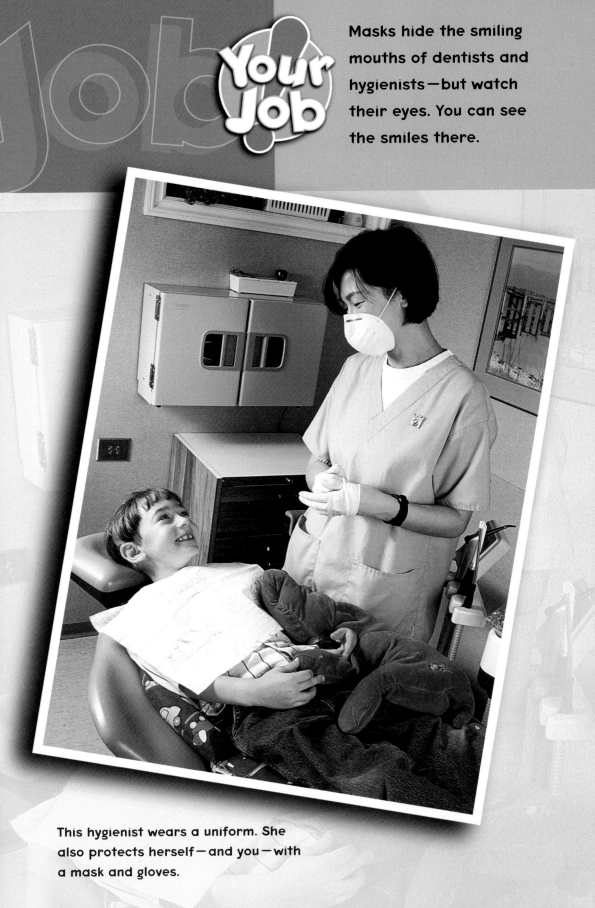

This hygienist wears a uniform. She also protects herself—and you—with a mask and gloves.

One Tooth, Two Teeth

Run a finger along your teeth—top and bottom. You can probably feel 20 to 24 of them. By the time you were two or three years old, you likely had all 20 of your primary teeth. They're also called baby, milk, or first teeth. At age six or seven, 4 permanent—or adult—teeth usually grow in behind these teeth. Other adult teeth soon start replacing the primary teeth.

Dentists examine your mouth to find out how your teeth are growing in. They feel the tops and sides of each tooth with a thin tool called an explorer. They check for any cracks or holes and see if your gums are firm and pink. A small mirror on a handle helps dentists peer into the hard-to-see parts of your mouth.

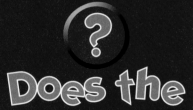

? Does the Explorer Bother Your Teeth or Gums?

The dentist moves it gently along all your teeth and gums. But a painful tooth or gum can feel sore if the explorer—or anything else—touches it. That's why it's best to get it fixed.

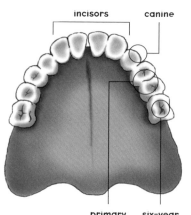

incisors · canine · primary molars · six-year molar

Compare this diagram with your own teeth. In each set—top and bottom—feel 4 incisors, 2 canines, and 4 primary molars. Have your six-year molars arrived yet?

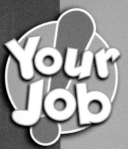

Hold your mouth open. You might also need to turn your head slightly. The dentist will tell you when.

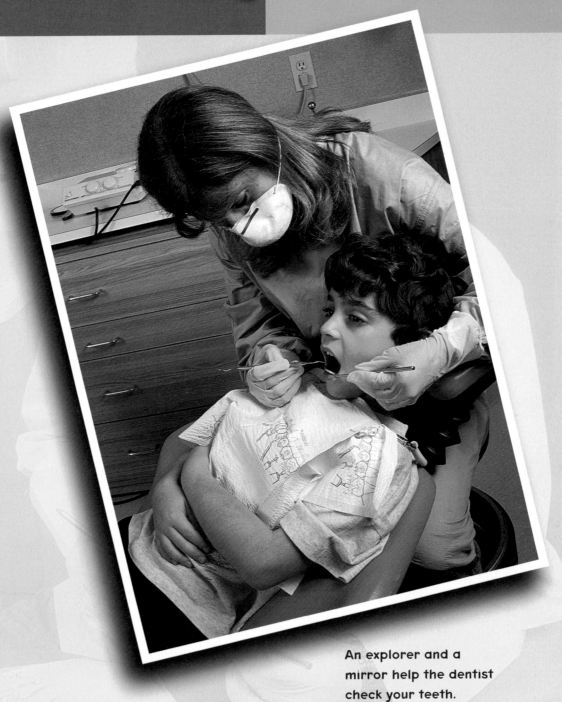

An explorer and a mirror help the dentist check your teeth.

Inside Look

Soon after you were born, adult teeth began forming in your jaws. Dentists check to see how these teeth are growing by looking at special photos. They use an X-ray machine — a camera that photographs insides, instead of outsides.

Holes, called cavities, that are too small to see with the eye show up on X-ray photos. So do cavities that form between teeth where the explorer can't search. Dentists try to find — and fix — them while they're still small.

For X-ray pictures, you wear a thick apron so only your jaws and teeth are photographed. The film usually goes inside your mouth in a plastic or cardboard holder. You clutch the holder between your top and bottom teeth.

Sometimes a different kind of X-ray camera is used to get all your teeth into one picture. It moves around you as it photographs — and you don't have to hold the film in your mouth.

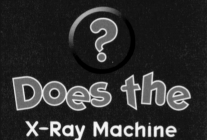

Does the X-Ray Machine Feel Odd?

It doesn't even touch you, but the apron feels heavy. If the film holder is at the back of your mouth, it might press into your gums or make you gag. Be brave — an X-ray takes only a few seconds.

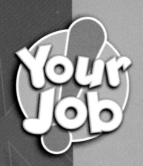

If you're given a film holder, grip it firmly. Hold still so the X-ray machine can get clear pictures. Then look at your X-ray photos, and ask your dentist to tell you what they show.

As you get ready to have your teeth X-rayed, a big apron covers most of your body.

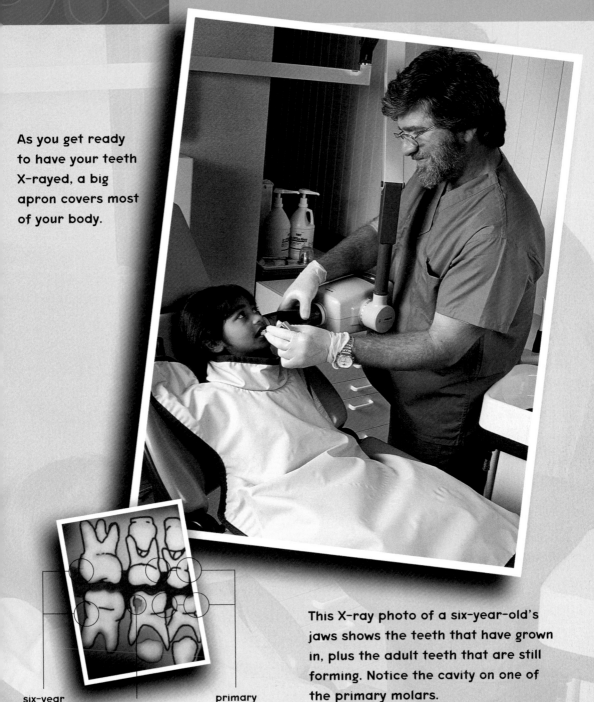

six-year molars

cavity

primary molars

This X-ray photo of a six-year-old's jaws shows the teeth that have grown in, plus the adult teeth that are still forming. Notice the cavity on one of the primary molars.

Clean-up Team

By brushing your teeth twice a day, you remove a lot of the germs that can cause cavities and sore gums. Still, you can't catch them all. A sticky layer of germs—plaque—is always forming on your teeth. Over time, it hardens into a tough coating called calculus or tartar, which you can't get off. That's why your teeth need a special cleaning when you visit the dentist.

Hygienists often scrape off calculus with a small tool called a scaler. Sometimes they also shake off the calculus with a tool that fits on the end of a narrow air hose. The hose powers many of the tools in a dentist's office. As hygienists remove the calculus, they rinse your mouth with water.

Next, they clean and polish your teeth with toothpaste and little tools that spin around on the end of the air hose. They remove any plaque that's still there and rinse out your mouth. The cleaning and polishing smooths your teeth, making it harder for plaque to stick to them.

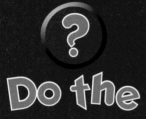

? Do the Cleaning Tools Bother Your Mouth?

They can tickle, and the whirring sound of the tools on the end of the air hose might surprise you. The toothpaste probably tastes different from what you use at home.

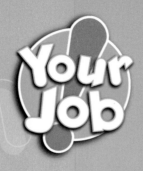

Opening your mouth wide makes it easier to reach some teeth, but harder to reach others. Work with the hygienist, spreading your jaws a lot—or a little—as needed. If asked, raise or lower your chin and turn your head from side to side.

Calculus has formed on the sides of this molar.

Calculus

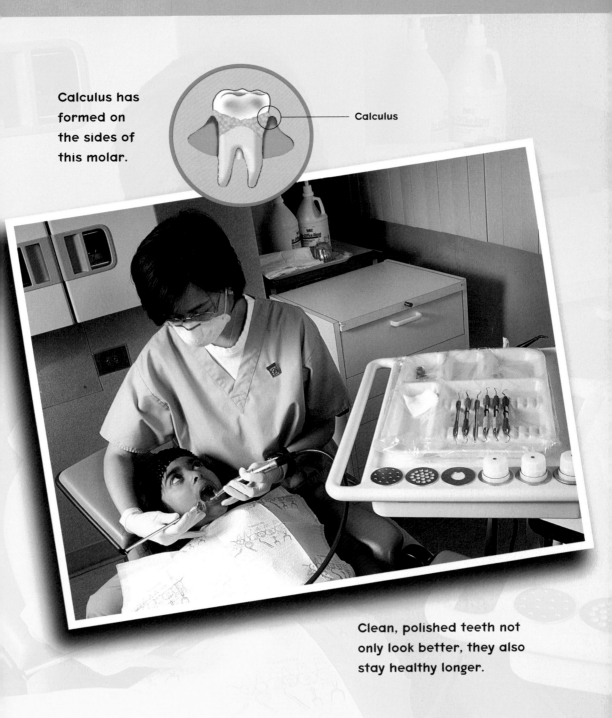

Clean, polished teeth not only look better, they also stay healthy longer.

Water Control

Your mouth can't hold all the water that hygienists use to rinse your teeth. They stop their cleaning from time to time and may ask you to spit into a small sink by your chair. Or they use a handy tool called a saliva ejector. It works like a mini vacuum cleaner, gently sucking up water and any extra saliva — spit. It also helps remove bits of leftover toothpaste.

The saliva ejector is attached to a narrow hose, and has a smooth tip at the other end. Only the tip goes in your mouth.

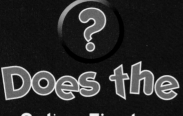

Does the Saliva Ejector Bother You?

No. It just makes gurgling sounds.

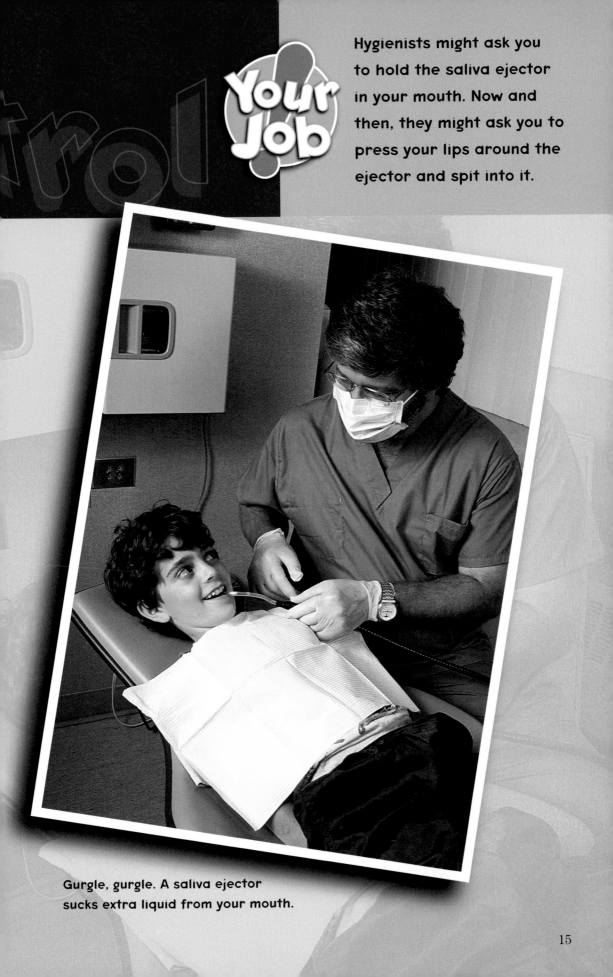

Hygienists might ask you to hold the saliva ejector in your mouth. Now and then, they might ask you to press your lips around the ejector and spit into it.

Gurgle, gurgle. A saliva ejector sucks extra liquid from your mouth.

Building Armor

Teeth grow their own armor — a hard outer layer called enamel. It's the hardest part of your body! Enamel helps protect teeth from germs that can cause cavities. Brushing with most toothpastes adds something called fluoride to your enamel. That makes the armor even tougher. So does taking fluoride pills or drinking water that has fluoride in it.

When you visit the dentist, you can get special fluoride treatments to strengthen your tooth enamel. Hygienists might paint your teeth with a liquid fluoride. They might put a fluoride gel or foam in holders that fit over your top and bottom teeth. Or they might ask you to swish some fluoride around in your mouth, then spit it out.

As the hygienists work, they use the saliva ejector to keep your mouth dry. Your enamel absorbs the fluoride — and don't worry: you can't see fluoride on your teeth. It's invisible.

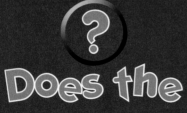

Does the Fluoride Treatment Bother Your Teeth?

The fluoride holders that fit over your teeth might feel a bit uncomfortable. Hang in. The treatment is soon over.

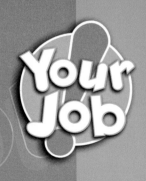

Fluoride comes in flavors such as cherry, mint—even bubble gum and butterscotch! Choose the one you like. After a treatment, wait for more than 30 minutes before eating or drinking. Some fluorides aren't good for your stomach.

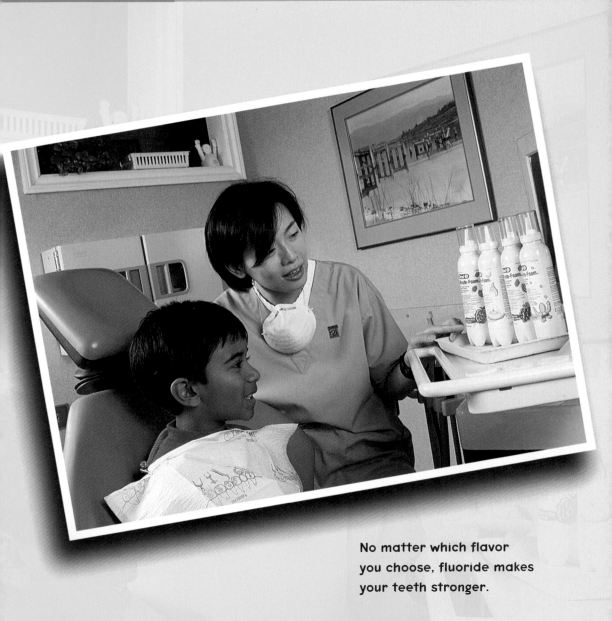

No matter which flavor you choose, fluoride makes your teeth stronger.

Sealing Out Trouble

S lide your tongue over your molars. Notice that the sides are smooth, but the chewing surfaces aren't. You can feel tiny pits and grooves that might trap germs, causing cavities.

Hygienists work to protect your molars by coating the chewing surfaces with a "sealant." It's a strong, see-through plastic.

They might first put a material on your teeth that helps the plastic stick. Then they rinse and dry the teeth before adding the sealant. They might also use a thin piece of rubber to keep your teeth dry. You'll read about this in "Get Ready" on page 22.

The sealant hardens in a few minutes—often on its own. But some kinds of sealants need help, so hygienists might shine a special light on your teeth for a few seconds.

Depending on what you chew and how you chew it, this tough coating might last two or three years. Then you can get another sealant on your teeth.

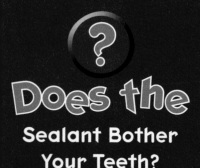

Does the
Sealant Bother Your Teeth?

Soon you won't even know it is there.

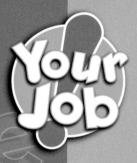

Your Job

Help the sealant last as long as possible by NOT chewing sticky stuff, ice cubes, or hard candy.

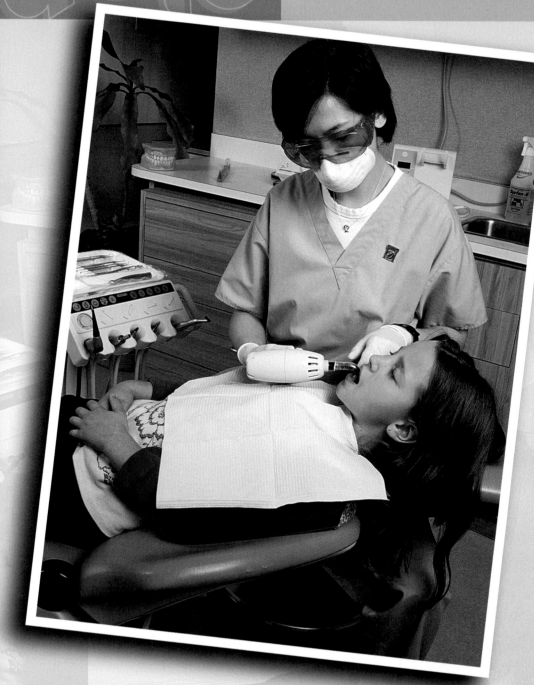

This hygienist uses light to harden sealant on molars.

Soothe a Tooth

If dentists find a cavity, they usually fix it before it gets bigger. Unless it's just a tiny hole, they often put the tooth to sleep before they work on it.

Dentists might spread a special liquid or gel on your gums or inside your cheek near the cavity. It makes the area around your tooth go numb — lose feeling — for a while. Then they might use a syringe, a tool with a tube and a hollow needle. Dentists place the tip of the needle in your gums or cheek. Liquid flows from the tube and out through the needle.

Some dentists prefer another method. Their offices may have a special high-powered tool that sprays liquid right into your gums or cheek near the cavity.

? Does the Syringe Bother Your Mouth?

If the dentist puts liquid or gel on your gums and cheek first, you shouldn't even feel the syringe. If not, you might feel it about as much as a hard pinch—but not for more than a second. As your tooth goes to sleep, your mouth might tingle and feel a bit strange.

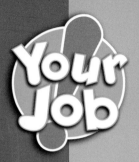

Your Job

Close your eyes and think about something you really like...a favorite game...your best friend... until the syringe is gone. Parts of your mouth, such as your cheek, tongue, lip, or gum, might feel numb for a while, so be careful not to bite them when you talk or chew.

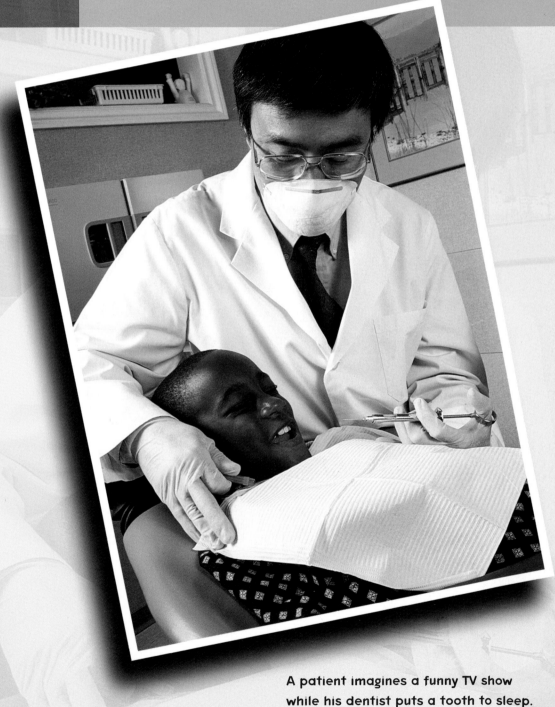

A patient imagines a funny TV show while his dentist puts a tooth to sleep.

Get Ready

Dentists must keep a tooth dry while they're fixing a cavity. Before they start work, they might place a few rolls of soft cotton near the tooth. The rolls soak up a lot of saliva.

Some dentists prefer to use a thin piece of rubber instead. They place it around the tooth that has a cavity. The rubber is stretched across a frame and attached to the tooth with a small clamp. It helps keep your wet tongue from touching the tooth. Then you don't have to spit out saliva while you're having your cavity mended — and the dentists don't need to use the saliva ejector as often.

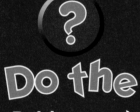

Do the
Rubber and the Clamp Bother Your Mouth?

They can make your mouth feel full. But some people feel less like gagging when dentists use the rubber and clamp to keep a tooth dry.

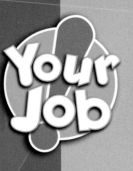

Your Job

Just for fun, think about all the other things people use to keep themselves dry...raincoats...boots... tents...

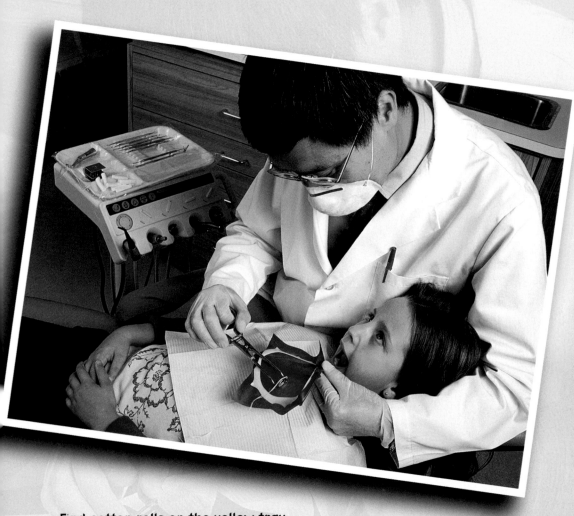

Find cotton rolls on the yellow tray. They help keep a tooth dry—just like the rubber that the dentist is putting in his patient's mouth.

Out with the Bad

Before dentists fill a cavity, they remove the parts of the tooth that germs have decayed. They often use a tool called a bur. It's powered by the same long air hose that runs many of their other tools.

When a bur spins fast against your tooth, it cleans out most of the decay. Sprays of water or air — or both — keep the tooth cool and flush away what the bur removes. Some dentists also have machines that use a special spray to dissolve decayed parts of the tooth.

Most dentists finish off by scooping out the last bits of decayed tooth with a tiny, narrow spoon.

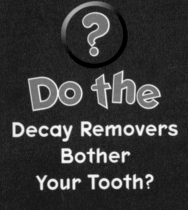

Do the Decay Removers Bother Your Tooth?

They can sound LOUD because the noise they make is inside your head, but they don't bother your tooth—it's asleep.

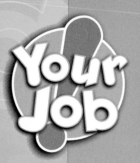

Your Job

Take deep, slow breaths. See how high you can count—in your head—before all the decay is removed from your tooth.

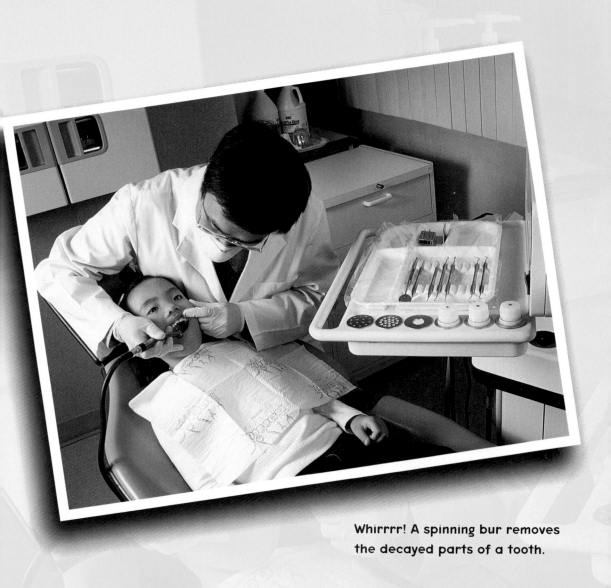

Whirrrr! A spinning bur removes the decayed parts of a tooth.

Get Set

After the decay is gone, dentists clean your tooth with sprays of water. Then they blow it dry with warm air from a narrow hose. They're careful not to leave trouble-causing germs behind when they fill in a hole.

If your cavity happens to be on the side of a tooth, dentists might wrap a thin collar around it. The collar works a bit like a jelly mold, holding a filling in place until set. Then the collar is removed.

? Does the Collar Bother Your Mouth?

No. It's only in your mouth for a few minutes.

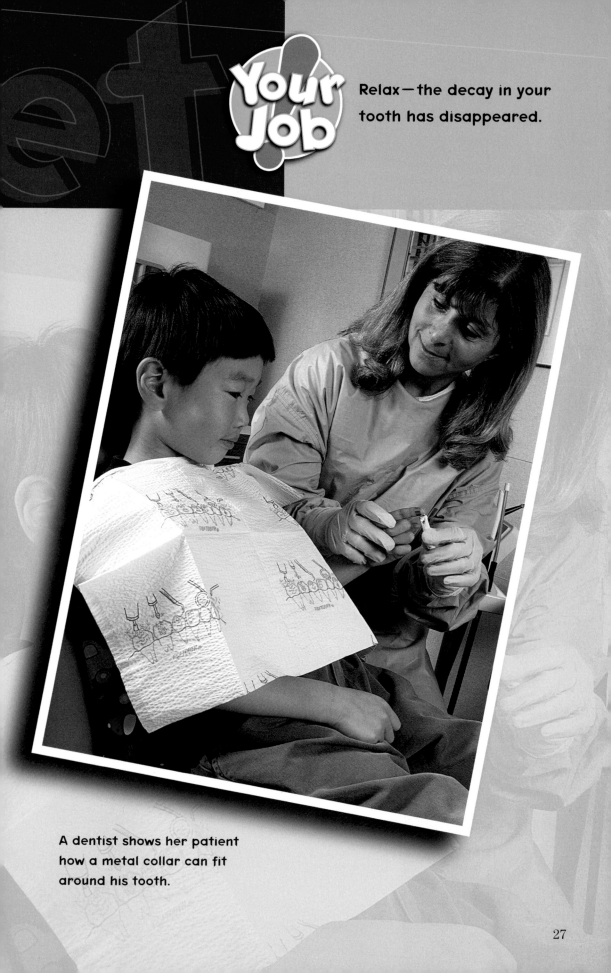

Your Job

Relax—the decay in your tooth has disappeared.

A dentist shows her patient how a metal collar can fit around his tooth.

In with the Good

To fix a hole in your tooth, dentists use a filling such as metal or plastic. They have different tools for different fillings — and for different teeth.

Dentists press a soft metal filling into a hole bit by bit. They shape it like the tooth and rub it smooth. The metal becomes solid after about an hour. But it usually takes a whole day to harden completely.

Plastic fillings are brushed on in layers that are hardened with a special light. Then dentists polish them with a disc that's powered by an air hose.

After you have a tooth fixed, you rinse your mouth with water, then spit. You check in a mirror to see your filling — and your great new smile. Done!

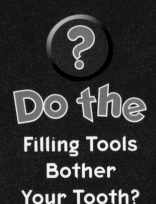

Do the

Filling Tools Bother Your Tooth?

No. Your tooth is still asleep.

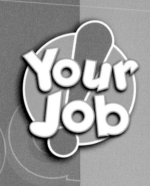

The dentist may ask you not to chew on a tooth that has a new filling—but only for a day or less. You might want to avoid food such as hot soup and ice cream for a while. Heat and cold can bother a newly filled tooth.

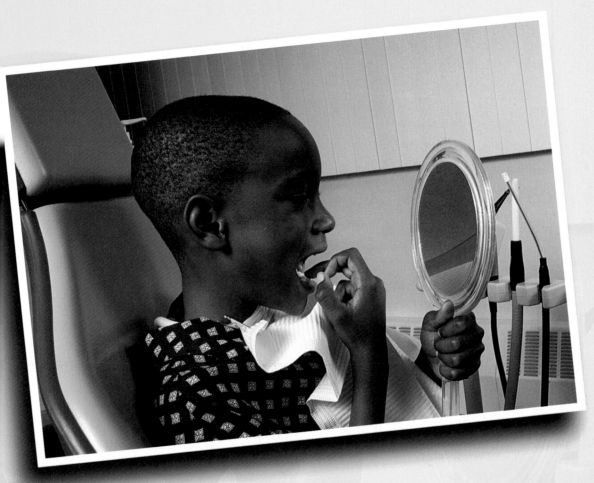

Check it out. A newly filled tooth looks and feels so much better than a decayed one.

Points for Parents

- Share this book with your children before they visit a dentist's office. It can reduce anxiety by helping them become familiar with the tools and treatments that dentists and hygienists use.
- Read the book out loud and study the pictures with your children. Encourage them to ask questions and discuss what they hear and see.
- Be open and honest in answering your children's questions and addressing their fears, but offer them no more information than you think they are ready to hear. Always stress the positive value of visiting a dentist.
- If you are uncomfortable — even fearful — about visiting a dentist yourself, be very careful not to display these feelings in words — or in body language!
- Ask your children how well they think the patients in the photos are doing their "jobs."
- Have your children find the toys that appear with these patients. Suggest they choose a toy of their own to bring with them on their visits to a dentist.
- Some children wrongly believe that dental visits are punishments for bad behavior. Watch for signs of such attitudes and reassure your children that the visits are solely about looking after their teeth.
- Stress the fact that dental visits are part of a normal, healthy routine for everybody.
- Contact the dentist's office ahead of time to learn its policy regarding parents accompanying their children into the treatment room. Some dentists prefer to have the parents in the room; others prefer not to.

After a visit to the dentist

- Praise your children for trying to do their special "jobs"— even if they might not have done them very well. Show your appreciation for the efforts they made and encourage them to try harder at the next visit.
- Review with your children any suggestions made during the visit about how they can care for their teeth better. Help them practice the teeth-cleaning procedures that the hygienist demonstrated. Stress that good care now can reduce problems later on.
- Reread this book with your children. Discuss how their dentist's tools compared to the ones you read about. Invite your children to ask questions about their visit.

Index

We acknowledge the support of the Canada Council for the Arts, the Ontario Arts Council, and the Government of Canada through the Book Publishing Industry Development Program (BPIDP) for our publishing activities.

Cataloging in Publication Data

Swanson, Diane, 1944–
  The dentist and you

Includes index.
ISBN 1-55037-729-9 (bound).—ISBN 1-55037-728-0 (pbk.)

1. Dentistry—Juvenile literature. 2. Children—Preparation for dental care—Juvenile literature. I. Title.

RK63.S92 2002   j617.6   C2001-903346-X

Photography by Warren Hales
Editing by Elizabeth McLean
Design by Irvin Cheung & Lisa Ma /iCheung Design
The text was typeset in ITC Century Book and Keedy Sans

Acknowledgments

Many wonderful people contributed greatly to the making of this book. For their dental expertise, sincerest thanks go to Dr. Bruce Yaholnitsky, Dr. Denise Carswell, and Dr. Frank Yung, who also made his office available for photographing. As well, the photo session was made possible by the enthusiastic cooperation of hygienist Florance Hui, several children from Charlton Public School and their parents, Susan Wilks—who helped out in so many ways, and keen photographer Warren Hales. Rick Wilks, Colleen MacMillan, Sandra Booth, and Elizabeth McLean pitched in to bring it all together. Thanks, everyone.

Published in the U.S.A. by
Annick Press (U.S.) Ltd.

Distributed in Canada by
Firefly Books Ltd.
3680 Victoria Park Avenue
Willowdale, ON
M2H 3K1

Distributed in the U.S.A. by
Firefly Books (U.S.) Inc.
P.O. Box 1338
Ellicott Station
Buffalo, NY 14205

Printed and bound in Canada.

Visit our website at **www.annickpress.com**